DAPOXETINE FOR MENS USAGE GUIDE

The In-depth Guide to Treat Premature Ejaculation, Fast Acting, Last Longer and Improved Sexual Satisfaction

Dr. Marcus Stone

Copyright © 2024 by Marcus, Stone

COPYRIGHT:

No part of this publication may be reproduced, stored in a retrieval system, or transmitted, in any form or by any means, electronic, mechanical, photocopying, recording, or otherwise, without the prior permission of the publisher.

DISCLAIMER:

The information provided in this book is intended for educational and informational purposes only. It is not intended as a substitute for professional medical advice, diagnosis, or treatment. Always seek the advice of your physician or other qualified health provider with any questions you may have regarding a medical condition.

Table of Contents

CHAPTER 1: 3

What is dapoxetine? 3

CHAPTER 2: 7

How the Body Absorbs It 7

CHAPTER 3: 17

Dosages and Administration 17

CHAPTER 4: 24

Contraindications (When It Should Not Be Used) 24

CHAPTER 5: 34

When to Take Dapoxetine? 34

THE END 42

CHAPTER 1:

What is dapoxetine?

Dapoxetine is primarily used to treat premature ejaculation in men. It is classified as a selective serotonin reuptake inhibitor (SSRI). Unlike other SSRIs, which are extensively used as antidepressants, dapoxetine has a fast onset of effect and is quickly removed from the body, making it ideal for on-demand therapy of premature ejaculation. It works by raising serotonin levels in the brain, which helps to delay and control ejaculation during sexual activity.

Dapoxetine's mechanism of action in the setting of premature ejaculation (PE) is based on its pharmacological features as a selective serotonin reuptake inhibitor (SSRI). Here's the breakdown:

Serotonin modulation: Serotonin is a neurotransmitter that plays a variety of physiological roles, including mood modulation and ejaculation control. Serotonin works in the brain's ejaculatory reflex pathway, affecting the timing of ejaculation.

Dapoxetine inhibits serotonin reuptake by neurons in the brain. This means that it prevents serotonin from being quickly reabsorbed by the presynaptic neuron when it is released into the synaptic cleft. Dapoxetine enhances the levels of serotonin in the synaptic cleft by reducing its reuptake.

Serotonin Activity: greater serotonin concentration in the synaptic cleft causes greater serotonin signaling. The increased serotonin activity alters the ejaculatory reflex circuit, causing a delay in the ejaculatory response.

Dapoxetine improves ejaculatory control by altering serotonin levels and brain activity. It prolongs the time it takes for ejaculation to occur, treating the primary symptom of premature ejaculation.

CHAPTER 2:

How the Body Absorbs It

The pharmacokinetics of Dapoxetine include its absorption, distribution, metabolism, and excretion processes. This is a thorough breakdown:

Absorption

Rapid Absorption: Dapoxetine is quickly absorbed following oral administration.

Peak plasma concentration (C_{max}) occurs roughly 1 to 2 hours after consumption.

Bioavailability: Dapoxetine has an absolute bioavailability of around 42%, which indicates that 42% of the orally delivered dose enters systemic circulation in an active state.

Distribution

Volume of Distribution: Dapoxetine has a large volume of distribution (about 162 liters), indicating that it is widely distributed throughout tissues.

Protein Binding: It is highly protein-bound (approximately

99%), particularly to plasma proteins like albumin and ?One-acid glycoprotein.

Metabolism

Dapoxetine is extensively metabolized in the liver via various pathways involving cytochrome P450 (CYP) enzymes, specifically CYP2D6 and CYP3A4.

Active and Inactive Metabolites: Dapoxetine's major metabolites are active and inactive. These metabolites have less pharmacological activity than the parent medication.

Excretion

Dapoxetine and its metabolites are eliminated by both the kidneys and the feces. Approximately 75% of an oral dose is eliminated in the urine, with the remainder excreted in the stool.

Dapoxetine has a relatively short elimination half-life, ranging from 1.5 to 2 hours. However, its active metabolites have a longer half-life, which contributes to its therapeutic efficacy.

Onset of Action: Because of its rapid absorption, this medication is most effective when given 1 to 3 hours before sexual activity.

Duration of Effect: Because of its short half-life, Dapoxetine is swiftly removed from the body, reducing long-term negative effects and making it suited for on-demand use.

Dapoxetine for Premature Ejaculation.

Dapoxetine is used primarily to treat premature ejaculation (PE). PE is a frequent sexual condition defined by the inability to regulate ejaculation, resulting in brief and unpleasant sexual sessions. Dapoxetine, a selective serotonin reuptake inhibitor (SSRI), increases serotonin levels in the brain. Serotonin is a neurotransmitter that regulates mood and behavior, as well as controlling ejaculation.

Dapoxetine is distinctive among SSRIs in that it has a fast onset of action and a short half-life, implying that it is swiftly absorbed and removed from the body. This makes it appropriate for usage as an on-demand medicine, administered one to three hours before sexual activity. Dapoxetine increases serotonin levels in the brain, which helps to delay ejaculation and allows men with PE to have more pleasurable sexual experiences.

It's vital to understand that dapoxetine isn't a cure for PE, but rather a medication that can help control it. It should be used as part of a complete PE management strategy that includes psychiatric counseling, behavioral approaches, and lifestyle changes. Furthermore, dapoxetine should be used under the supervision of a healthcare expert, as it may not be appropriate for everyone and may cause side effects or interactions with other drugs.

1 Efficacy

Dapoxetine has been demonstrated to be an effective treatment for premature ejaculation (PE). Clinical investigations and studies have proved its usefulness in enhancing multiple elements of sexual function:

Increased Intravaginal Ejaculatory Latency Time (IELT): Dapoxetine considerably delays ejaculation. According to studies, males who take Dapoxetine have a 2-3 times higher IELT than those who take a placebo.

Men claim having better control over ejaculation when taking Dapoxetine.

Dapoxetine improves sexual satisfaction for both men and their partners.

Patient-reported Outcomes: Surveys and surveys show that there is less distress associated with PE, more relationship satisfaction, and an overall higher quality of life.

CHAPTER 3:

Dosages and Administration

The suggested initial dose of Dapoxetine is 30 mg, administered 1 to 3 hours before sexual activity.

Dose Adjustment: The dose can be adjusted to a maximum of 60 mg if it is effective and well tolerated. This decision should be taken in conjunction with a medical professional.

Dapoxetine should not be taken more than once each 24-hour period.

Administration: Swallow the tablet whole, with a full glass of water. It can be taken with or without food, however high-fat meals may cause a minor delay in action.

Considerations: Before prescribing Dapoxetine, a complete medical history and examination should be performed to rule out any underlying disorders and ensure that the patient is a good candidate for the medicine.

Safety and tolerability

Common Side Effects:

Nausea is the most commonly reported adverse effect, affecting a considerable majority of users.

Dizziness: Patients may feel light-headed or dizzy, especially with the first dose.

Headache: Common, but typically mild to moderate in intensity.

Diarrhea is one of the gastrointestinal problems that have been documented.

Insomnia: Some people may have difficulties sleeping.

Serious side effects.

Syncope: A brief loss of consciousness, commonly caused by orthostatic hypotension (a quick drop in blood pressure when rising up).

Mood Changes: As with other SSRIs, there is a risk of mood changes, such as depression and suicide ideation, although these are uncommon.

Cardiovascular Events: Because dapoxetine might impact heart rate and blood pressure, persons with cardiovascular disorders should use it with caution.

Contraindications

Dapoxetine should not be used by people who have serious heart problems, such as heart failure, conduction abnormalities, or substantial ischemic heart disease.

It is not recommended for persons with moderate to severe liver impairment.

Dapoxetine may interact negatively with monoamine oxidase inhibitors and other serotonergic medications when used concurrently.

Known Hypersensitivity: If you have ever had an allergic reaction to Dapoxetine or its components, you should avoid using it.

Tolerability

Gradual Titration: Begin with a lower dose of 30 mg to assess tolerance and reduce adverse effects.

Patient Monitoring: It is recommended that patients have regular follow-ups to check adverse effects and change dosage as needed.

Education and Counseling: Patients should be informed about potential adverse effects and given guidance on how to manage them.

CHAPTER 4:

Contraindications (When It Should Not Be Used)

Counterindications

Dapoxetine should not be used in some instances because it has the potential for substantial side effects or a lack of efficacy. Here are the major contraindications:

Dapoxetine is contraindicated in persons with serious cardiovascular problems, including:

History of heart failure.

Conduction anomalies (for example, atrioventricular block)

Ischemic heart disease (angina, myocardial infarction)

Unstable hypertension or hypotension.

Syncope or Orthostatic Hypotension

Dapoxetine is not recommended for patients with moderate to severe liver impairment (Child-Pugh Class B and C).

Concomitant Use with Monoamine Oxidase Inhibitors (MAOIs): Due to the risk of serotonin syndrome, dapoxetine should not be administered concurrently or within 14 days of discontinuing MAOI treatment.

Individuals who have a known hypersensitivity to Dapoxetine or any of its components should avoid using the medicine.

Drug Interactions.

Dapoxetine may interact with other drugs, reducing their efficacy or increasing the risk of side effects. Here are some important medication interactions:

Monoamine Oxidase Inhibitors (MAOIs): Taking Dapoxetine concurrently with MAOIs or within 14 days after stopping MAOIs might result in serotonin syndrome, which includes symptoms like agitation, hallucinations, hyperthermia, tremors, and coma.

Serotonergic medications: Due to the potential of serotonin syndrome, dapoxetine should be used with caution when combined with other serotonergic medications such as SSRIs, SNRIs, tricyclic antidepressants, triptans, and some opioids.

CYP3A4 Inhibitors: Drugs that block the CYP3A4 enzyme, such as ketoconazole, ritonavir, and clarithromycin, can raise Dapoxetine plasma levels, thus increasing the risk of side effects.

CYP2D6 Inhibitors: Taking powerful CYP2D6 inhibitors (such as quinidine, fluoxetine, or paroxetine) concurrently can increase Dapoxetine exposure, increasing the risk of side effects.

Dapoxetine may enhance the hypotensive effects of alpha-blockers and antihypertensive drugs, resulting in orthostatic hypotension and syncope. Combining these drugs should be done with caution.

Alcohol consumption should be limited or avoided while taking Dapoxetine since it has the potential to aggravate central nervous system depression and impair cognitive and motor performance.

Side Effects:

Some people may experience side effects from dapoxetine, as with any other medicine. Here are some common negative effects related with dapoxetine:

Nausea is one of the most common side effects of Dapoxetine. It may occur immediately after taking the medicine and might be mild to moderate in severity.

Dizziness or light-headedness may develop, particularly when getting up suddenly from a sitting or laying posture. This adverse effect is typically temporary and improves with continuing use.

Headache: Dapoxetine users frequently report headaches. They are usually mild to moderate in intensity and can improve over time or with symptomatic therapy.

Diarrhea: Diarrhea is a possible adverse effect of Dapoxetine. This gastrointestinal ailment is typically moderate and temporary.

Insomnia: Some people may experience difficulty falling and staying asleep. It is best to take Dapoxetine early in the day to reduce the chance of sleeplessness.

Dapoxetine may also cause weariness. This may occur, particularly in the early phases of treatment, but it usually improves with continuing use.

Dapoxetine users have complained dry mouth. Staying hydrated and eating sugar-free gum or candy may assist with this symptom.

Decreased Libido: Dapoxetine may cause a decrease in sexual desire or libido. This can cause distress for certain individuals, however it is usually very transient.

Perspiration: Some people who use Dapoxetine have noticed excessive perspiration or diaphoresis. This side effect is typically moderate and may not necessitate action.

Blurred vision or visual abnormalities might develop in rare circumstances.

CHAPTER 5:

When to Take Dapoxetine?

Dapoxetine is normally taken as needed, just before planned sexual activity. Here are some guidelines about when to take Dapoxetine.

Timing: Dapoxetine should be taken about 1 to 3 hours before sexual activity. This scheduling permits the medicine to reach peak plasma concentrations and take effect when needed.

On-Demand usage: Unlike certain drugs that require daily dose Dapoxetine is intended for usage on demand. This means that you only take it when you intend to engage in sexual behavior.

Flexible arranging: Dapoxetine allows for more freedom in arranging sexual activities because it does not have to be taken at the same time every day. You can take it if you and your partner intend to be intimate.

Food Consideration: Dapoxetine may be taken with or without food. However, high-fat meals may cause a minor delay in the commencement of effect, so avoid heavy meals if feasible.

Individual Response: The appropriate timing of Dapoxetine may differ depending on individual parameters such as metabolism, tolerance, and sexual circumstances. It may take some experimentation to determine the ideal timing for you.

Dosage Adjustment: If the initial dose of Dapoxetine (usually 30 mg) does not produce the intended effect, you may consult with your healthcare professional about increasing the dosage to 60 mg, as long as it is safe and acceptable for you.

Here's an overview of the main aspects concerning Dapoxetine:

Dapoxetine is a short-acting selective serotonin reuptake inhibitor (SSRI) that is primarily used to treat premature ejaculation in men.

Mechanism of Action: It operates by blocking the serotonin transporter, resulting in higher serotonin levels in the synaptic cleft and delaying ejaculation through neurotransmission.

Pharmacokinetics: Dapoxetine is quickly absorbed after oral administration, achieves peak plasma concentration in 1 to 2 hours, has a large volume of distribution, is extensively metabolized in the liver, and has a short elimination half-life of 1.5 to 2 hours.

Efficacy: Dapoxetine prolongs intravaginal ejaculatory latency time (IELT), improves ejaculatory control, increases sexual satisfaction, and has a positive impact on PE-related patient outcomes.

Dosage and Administration: It is taken as needed, 1 to 3 hours before sexual activity, with a starting dose of 30 mg that can be increased to a maximum of 60 mg based on efficacy and tolerability.

Tolerance and safety: Common adverse effects include nausea, dizziness, headache, diarrhea, sleeplessness, and exhaustion. Serious side effects include syncope, mood swings, and cardiovascular problems. Individuals with substantial cardiovascular issues, liver impairment, concurrent use of MAOIs, or hypersensitivity to the medicine should not take dapoxetine.

Drug Interactions: Dapoxetine may interact with MAOIs, serotonergic medications, CYP3A4 inhibitors, CYP2D6 inhibitors, alpha-blockers, antihypertensive medicines, and alcohol, potentially causing side effects or decreased efficacy.

When to Take: Dapoxetine is taken 1 to 3 hours before planned sexual activity, providing scheduling flexibility and enabling for on-demand use.

THE END

www.ingramcontent.com/pod-product-compliance
Lightning Source LLC
Chambersburg PA
CBHW050029230526
45470CB00003B/1197